Like Joy

Like Joy

Glenna Cook

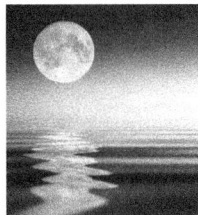

MoonPath Press

Poetry
ISBN 978-1-936657-88-9

Cover art: *Bird and Flowers,*
Photographed and processed by Lyn Marie Wells

Author photo by Jim and Ginny Christensen

Book design by Tonya Namura, using Kristi (display)
and Garamond Premier Pro (text)

MoonPath Press, an imprint of Concrete Wolf Poetry Series,
is dedicated to publishing the finest poets
living in the U.S. Pacific Northwest.

MoonPath Press
c/o Concrete Wolf
PO Box 2220
Newport, OR 97365-0163

MoonPathPress@gmail.com

http://MoonPathPress.com

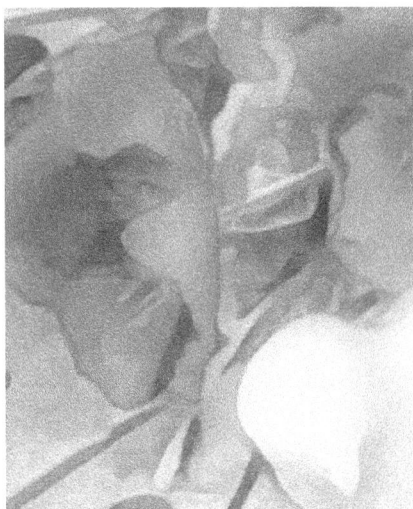

Dedicated to
my son, Ralph,
who is also a Parkinson's Warrior,
and my daughter, Lyn,
who is there for me when I need her.

Table of Contents

The Art of Being a Healing Presence

Like Joy

Mr. Parkinson

A Poem of Hope and Faith

Nothing that is worth doing can be
achieved in a lifetime; therefore,
we must be saved by hope. Nothing
which is true or beautiful or good
makes complete sense in any immediate
context in history; therefore, we must be
saved by faith.
                —*Reinhold Niebuhr*

Like a free-flowing river
my day dawns with hope's
promise of a poem, true
beautiful and good.
No more obstacles the size
of elephants blocking the path
toward my goal. No more
procrastination. No more distractions
snaking through my brain.
No more prickly judgements
shrinking my confidence.
Eyes open, I breathe in love,
breathe out foggy blindness,
and call upon my muse for help.
Pushing hard against the blockade
of fear, I let my pen flow like
a river. The rhythm swings
the cadence sings a song
of life that never ends.

New Friend

At the art museum,
two hours spent filling
my eyes with imagery,
I become aware
of your insistent presence.
My right hand,
resting in the crook of my left arm,
begins to tremble.
My gait concedes
to a slight unsteadiness.

I have decided to love you,
a part of me I didn't ask for
but won't reject
now that I know you're not leaving.

You even serve a purpose,
sending me places I may otherwise
be too lazy to go
if I didn't feel your tug.

Last week, I walked along Ruston Way,
felt the cool breeze coming off
the water on a hot afternoon.

Wednesday, I met a friend for lunch.

Today, I'm here.
You'll be my incentive
to fill my days
with nourishing pursuits,
reminding me,
that each moment I'm alive
I can choose to be grateful.

When things happen unexpectedly—

a dark wind blowing me off course
without a compass or words spoken
from an unknown source to guide me.

If I forget to be scared,
I'll look within and follow
my North Star through uncharted
waters to a new destination.

I can't always stroll in an orchard
of bliss. To live a rich life, I must
stretch toward the unease
of uncertainties never explored.

That tarantula walking
across my path might be a threat
or an opportunity to face
an unfounded fear.

The Dizzying Pleasure of Sniffing

My first symptom of Parkinson's
was losing my sense of smell.
This has its downside
but some advantages, too.

I'm not bothered by the rancid
stink of a person or dog that needs
a bath. That means I don't know
when I need one, either.
If people move to the far
side of the elevator when I get on,
that's a clear indication that I do.

Luckily, my nose is selective
in what it excludes. I can smell
the acrid odor of smoke
and a few foul chemical
pungencies that signal danger.

Bacon. I fiercely miss the friendly
smell of bacon. A BLT
doesn't even tempt me anymore.
Tangerine's clean sharp scent—gone.
The exotic perfume of jasmine,
heavy sweetness of lilac, delicate
seduction of a rose—gone.

I can't smell ozone rising
from the ground after a long
sought-after rain. Butter and
dill weed on new potatoes—
how I miss that country comfort.

I see a kite in the shape of a fly
flying high, a grandfather
and his progeny running to make it
fly higher, and my mind recalls
the dizzying pleasure of sniffing
sheets dried on a line on a windy day.

Affliction

Are you my enemy or my friend?

You set boundaries to keep me in my place,
yet challenge me to claim my destiny.

Constrained by your defining terms,
boundaries you've set to keep me in my place,

I'll wrestle with you for my right to be
uncontained within defining terms.

I challenge you and claim my destiny.

I'll wrestle you until I come to be
your limping enemy, your victorious friend.

Mr. Parkinson

                I
Parkinson's,
the progressive, neurological disease
that bears your name
appears in my body as in no other.
Like snowflakes,
no one's mix, from a multitude
of symptoms, is the same.
So far, there is no known cure.

In some cases, you are inherited.
A long time ago,
you took down my beloved
Aunt Fern, and you have
invaded the body
of Ralph, my beloved son.

My grandson, Chad, may have you
from exposure to burn pits
during the Afghanistan war.
Agent Orange gave you to troops
in Vietnam. Toxic chemicals
can be anywhere in this polluted
world—in our food supply,
our water, our air.

You may have claimed me years ago
when I lost my sense of smell,
a common early symptom.
You won that round, Mr. Parkinson.
I said goodbye
to the flavor of a raspberry.
Now it's only a sweet and tart, seedy
morsel. I treasure the bitterness

of black coffee, dark chocolate.
I miss the scent of a rose, lilacs,
a baby's skin, bread baking.
Scents evoke emotions.
My emotions are flat. How do you
compensate for that, Mr. Parkinson?

            II
You are so subtle, Mr. Parkinson.
You started with a slight tremor in my right
hand, then a slower step
when I was tired. Nothing to worry about.
You wanted me to wait until
you got a good hold on me.

My neurologist, a movement disorder
specialist, prescribed dopamine pills,
told me to exercise. I have done
Peddling for Parkinson's,
Rock Steady Boxing, Ai-Chi and Tai-chi,
water aerobics, weight classes,
Dance for PD, pole-hiking and yoga.

The tremors subsided.
My movements improved.
I have this, I said to myself,
and to you. But for how long?

I work to stay fit, because I know,
if I skip exercise, you will be right there
giving me your tight, rigid muscles.
It will hurt to walk or stand straight,
so I will take shorter steps, bend
over a little. That is how you take
hold and progress—tight

muscles, less movement, less
movement, tighter muscles.
If I allow the cycle to continue
I will soon walk stooped behind a walker,
shuffling along. Now I know to walk
through the pain, stretch my muscles,
take big steps, stand up straight.
I am aware that it would take
only one fall, one broken bone,
to put me out of commission,
shut down my exercise.
I'll face that, if it comes
and you will see,
I still won't give up.

III

It's not enough that you want to affect
every muscle in my body, even those that
control eye focus, elimination, speech and
facial expression. No, you have a higher goal.
You want my mind, my mood, my emotions.

I feel neither ecstatic joy or deep sorrow.
I know when I am happy or sad.
My mind tells me so.
As I taste raspberry, I taste life, but the flavor
which gives me the highs and lows
of living it is compromised.

When my oldest son died from cancer, I barely cried.
When my husband died, it was the same.
When pressure mounted to let my feelings out,
I binged on sci-fi, fantasy books,
or *Gilmore Girls* on Netflix.
Or I curled into a ball and took a nap.

My therapist prescribed antidepressants
and I survived. When depression failed
to bring me down, you brought out your
strongest weapon—Apathy.

Apathy just doesn't care. Apathy checks out
and lets you win.
Here's where I go to the mat with you.
Here's where I bring out my strongest weapon—
my mind's ability to choose.

I choose, Mr. Parkinson, to resist
your persistent, seductive desire
for me to retreat from the world and give up.
I will fight with you, until the end
because I choose to be strong
and I choose to be happy.

Depression

A thick gray blanket
wraps me, holds me inside
its soft cocoon.

I know I must struggle
against its seduction,
connect with the outside world.

Inwardness can be good,
can make one wise.
Not within the gray blanket.

Inwardness must be able
to breathe in and breathe out.
This blanket suffocates.

Survivor's Remorse

For Daryl

Mr. Parkinson, I'm so angry!
Why, why did you treat Daryl so brutally?
Did he not follow your protocol
religiously enough?

He was a religious man himself,
a pastor of a lively congregation
who loved him. A strong
well-built man, beautiful as a tiger
with a voice clear as a trombone,
words spilling out of his mouth like music.

How did he become a target for your
entropy? You were an opposing force
taking down his life force, ignoring
the first law of thermodynamics:

Energy can be neither created nor destroyed.

Daryl had energy, and you destroyed it.

I saw it all. He once asked me, *Is there any
hope that I will get better?* I had to tell him
that his best hope was to work hard
toward not getting worse.

The company one keeps seeps deep.
When you latched onto him, Mr. Parkinson,
the voice that sang those beautiful hymns
began to sing the blues.

It takes one to know one, and I know you
to be a cruel and heartless taskmaster,
as am I, as I force myself to slavishly follow
your rules to keep myself functioning, while
I uselessly watch your victims
lose all hope and sink
into your greedy, waiting arms.

The Truth of the Matter

Mr. Parkinson, you say
you want me to be your friend.
I would escape the hold you have on me.
You discipline me constantly.
I'm tired of your control.

Every three hours, throughout every day,
you remind me to take a pill.
You make me watch every step I take
or you throw me off-balance.
If I fail to move my body
to meet your expectation,
you give me pain. You tell me
what foods to eat or not eat.
You insist that I socialize
or you sink me in depression.

You have hung around too long.
I want to be free of you
but you refuse to let me go.

The truth of the matter is,
like it or not, I'll do as you say.
I have little choice.
It's wiser to obey you
than to be your enemy.

All Things Must End

These last golden rays of September
will give way to darker,
colder, more turbulent skies.

Every season holds
hints of the final season.
Each new beginning dawns
more tenuously.
Each year finds me more alone,
left behind to live
with ghostly memories
of those I loved.

Time slows; a quiet lethargy descends.
The incoming tide grows slack,
gives in to the moon's persistent pull.
Should I give in
or resist the undertow?

In the still-dark hours of morning
I push myself out of bed,
swallow a battery of pills,
eat a healthy breakfast,
oatmeal and a fruit smoothie,
then go to the Pedaling for
Parkinson's class at the YMCA.

Eighty to ninety RPMs,
forty-five minutes
three times a week,
champions of the stationary bike,
pedaling for our lives.

About Losing and Meaning

My most boring task is sorting
through my ego for something
I've lost that I never needed anyway.

Sorting through my mind for something
lost, because I forgot I needed it,
I find my favorite cellist,
Yo-Yo Ma, a man whose ego
never got in the way of pleasing me
with his music. I heard
he forgot his cello in the back
of a taxi. He thought that was funny.

What could I lose that would
mean as much to me as Yo-Yo Ma's
cello means to him, and could I laugh
if I forgot it? Of course, he laughed
with relief when he found it again.

What if I forgot how to write a poem,
or write anything, or even how to think
about writing? Is my meaning tied to
whether I can write? I see plenty
of people around me every day
who have forgotten how to write.
Some have even forgotten how to laugh.

I haven't forgotten how to laugh.

Like Joy

I sit at the edge of my bed
resisting the urge to climb back in
and ask myself the familiar question,
Will I ever again feel joy?

From my radio a guitarist
strums a song so uplifting
I rise to my feet and sway
my body in a dance.

My arms lift and fall
in waves and circles.
My feet know
just where to step
in rhythm to the tender
notes of the plucked strings.

My balance is perfect.
No sign of Parkinson's.
How strange.

On and on, the music
moves me in graceful motion,
loses me in time.

Do I feel joy?
Not the exhilarating,
gut-quivering excitement
I used to know.

Yet, at this moment
I experience in my body
an exquisite, inexplicable
lightness of being.

When I Fly

God, I meet you in my quiet place.
I come with noisy, troubled mind.
You comfort my confusion and distress.
Bear me up as I grow weary.
Still the noisy static of my mind.
Where will I go when I fly from this body,
after it has grown too weary?
Comfort my confusion and distress.
Say that when I fly from this old body,
you'll meet me in a quiet place.

Memories

An Unresolved Riddle

What we don't understand as innocent
children, sometimes reveals itself
in our more seasoned musings
when experience adds context
to memories as they surface
with their troublesome questions.

Memory can play tricks on us
but so can forgetting.
The more we give room
for imagination to embellish
our stories, the more
metaphors insist
on peeking from behind the curtain
of our denial.

Myth can tell more truth
than rationality, and just
because the facts may not
resemble what we remember
doesn't mean it isn't true.

First Grade Love

First day of school
out on the playground
under the cold, steel monkey bars
Joe said I was his girlfriend.

No, I'm not!

      Yes, you are!

No, I'm not!

And I ran away.

Joe, with his straight, brown hair
falling over his glass-green eyes,
Joe, with his grass-stained knees,
Joe, with his laugh that sounded
like water spilling over rocks,
Joe, with a smile that showed off
his shining, white teeth
too big for his mouth,
Joe, that smelled like an autumn
breeze and a cow barn.

I thought I could play hard to get.
I thought Joe would try harder
to win me. Every day
Joe had a new girlfriend.

Waking Up After an Ice Storm

The world is bathed in crystal,
radiant under a bright blue sky.
Every tree and bush, every branch,
twig, and needle, every blade of grass,
glitters in the brittle, cold light.

Listen.

In the morning's silence,
I think I hear their soft
tinkling chimes in the playful
caress of the wind.

No one walks about on the slippery
paths or drives on the treacherous roads.
Robins fluff their feathers for warmth.
In their burrows, small animals nestle
against each other and sleep.

We hunker down in our safe, cozy
houses, hope the power stays on,
say to ourselves, *This too shall pass.*

Such rare beauty seldom lingers.

Watching Bears

Once, when I was eight, my brother ten,
Dad let us ride with him in his company's
eighteen-wheeler, to Forks, a tiny town
near the National Rain Forest on the Olympic
Peninsula, to deliver a load of lumber.

On the way home, driving through
foothills of the Olympic Range,
my father suddenly exclaimed,

Look at that!

He pulled up at the side of the road,
grabbed binoculars from under the seat
and scrambled out of the truck. We followed
to see what he saw that amazed him.

Far up the mountain, clambering
over a mess of clear-cut forestland
two huge bears, one brown, one black
were foraging, probably for blackberries
that thrived in the liberated sunlight
among the stumps and discarded debris.

They were not aware of us,
or if they were, didn't care.
Dad and Brother spoke
in voices hushed with awe.
I was scared.

I had never seen real bears before,
except when they chased me in nightmares.
I didn't know how fast they could cover

the distance between us. I scurried
into the truck and huddled in worry
until the bears ambled away and we left.

Not the first time, or the last, I let
fear come between me and life's adventures.

She Named Her Wheelchair Nadine

Rather a friend
than an embarrassment.

Easier to laugh with her than cry
when the cruel boys pushed them

off the sidewalk during trick-or-treat.
She pretended she and Nadine

were evil witches, and together they cast
a ghastly curse on those nasty boys.

The thing is

to love a rainy day in the darkest month,
huge drops making a drizzly, mournful
sound, takes a childhood memory:
my brother and I pulling on boots
and wading in the pond
in our front lawn, formed by a week's
overabundance of downpour.
In our minds, we're walking
in the surf at the ocean beach.

To love this old quilt, frayed in spots,
that still covers me under the blue-
flowered comforter on my bed,
takes some imagination.
The bright and not-so-bright
pieces of fabric that form the circles
of the pattern, were once leftover
scraps of housedresses and men's shirts,
petticoats and pinafores, aprons and nighties,
Sunday best and everyday work clothes,
curtains and school clothes, bibs and
baby clothes, pajamas and potholders,

sewn by mothers and grandmothers,
the quilt itself made by women at the
church mission circle, priced to sell
by how many spools of thread
it took to quilt it.

Under it, I feel the soothing
weight of time and age,
life lived hard and simply.
When I die, I wish to be wrapped in it.

One Summer Morning in My Woods

The sun, risen after a radiant dawn,
filters green light through
vine maple leaves. I lie
dreamlike on a mossy log,
back of my head cradled
in my hands, thinking I'm in Paradise.

I hear a buzz and looking up
see a hummingbird drinking nectar
from honeysuckle blossoms.

Frightened, I run home to tell
my parents of the biggest
bumble bee I ever saw.

The First Man on the Moon

I watched like a high school roadie
as he stepped out of the magic
moon chariot. No one ever thought it
possible, yet footprints don't lie.

He walked a bubblegum gait
bouncing a jig like treading
on air, except there was no air,
only moon space.

You and I played telephone tag,
each wanting to be first to tell
the other, the world had widened.

A Cure for the Housing Problem

A few years ago,
in one day
a work crew built
a tiny house
in my neighbors'
backyard.

It was for Grandma
because Grandpa
had died recently.

They built it right next
to the trampoline
on which
two little kids,
Olive and Mosby,
jumped every day,
their curly blond
heads rising above
the fence. They
would wave at me
then disappear
only to bounce
back up again.

It seemed to me
back then
a splendid idea
to populate
backyards
with tiny houses.

I wish I could go back in time

to walk with you
as a daughter and a friend
and listen
as you tell me
of your deferred dreams
that never came to pass.

How you put aside
your own needs
to meet the needs of others
suppressing disappointment,
telling yourself your dreams
were not as important.

I wish I could tell you
in this new time dimension,
having lived through
my own struggles,
that now I understand
how much you sacrificed
for me so that I could have
what you did not.

I appreciate
as I didn't then, how much
you gave up, how little
you sought in return.
How sometimes at night
your tired body ached with need,
and you cried silent tears
into your pillow.

Three Women

Three women in the photo on my phone.
Three generations: daughter, mother,
grandmother.

At forty, the daughter still blooms
with youthful beauty. Her skin,
smooth as a rose petal,
shows little sign of facing
life's cruelest challenges.
She still thrives on the illusion
that someday she can make
all her troubles disappear
and will one day gain
all she dreams of attaining.

At sixty-six, the mother,
beautiful as a full-blown rose,
colors her long hair blond. She shows
worry-wrinkles between her eyebrows
and at the corners of her eyes.
She has survived hard times
and disillusionments, has learned
that no one's life is free of pain
and some dreams must be relinquished.

At eighty-seven, the grandmother
wears her gray hair short.
The only beauty in her furrowed face
streams from smiling eyes
full of love for the other two. She knows
she will leave them and accepts this,
as they do not. She has shed her illusions
and rests in the knowledge
that she can change nothing of her past,

almost nothing in the course to come
and has only each present day,
in which to live well.

Love's Acquiescence

Behind the curtain of my mind
lives a memory
wrapped in tissue paper,
precious as a kiss.

It doesn't begin where
you left off. It starts
where we began when you
promised you would always
remember me young.

I aged. So did you.
Neither of us saw it coming.
As the years slipped by,
only a softer tolerance
of change and decay,
a weathering of resistance.

A piano plays in the background,
pleasing to the ear.

My Little Blue Bird

On top of the bookcase
that holds my poetry
perches a small, glass bird
blue as a cloudless sky
holding its tail high
as if singing.

In the seventies I bought it
from a little gift shop
long since closed
that specialized in Fenton glassware.

In 1905, the year my mother was born,
two brothers, Frank and John,
started the Fenton Art Glass Company.

They built their factory
in Williamstown, West Virginia.
In 2011, having served
its family well, it closed.
Now, another company
with bigger capacity
uses its methods of molding
and Williamstown Elementary
sits on the site
where the factory stood.

Frank and John
would have liked that.

Little Blue Bird has become
a collectors' item, valued in
gift shops, online and at auctions.
I don't care about that.

I just love that it's pretty,
that it has graced my poetry
bookshelves all these years
and that now
it exists in this poem.

Wonder

Once as a young girl,
I followed the creek until
I came upon a small pond
I didn't know was there,
hidden among the Douglas firs.
I claimed it as my own and
went there often to wonder.

In this quiet sanctuary,
I felt like my true self.

I know a man who received
a profound sense of himself
when he ran along a beach
and perceived a whale beyond the surf
swimming along with him.

What do you feel when you see
the first falling star of the summer
in a navy-blue sky?

Wake up!
You are surrounded by marvels
that could astound you.
Claim them for your own
and let them change you.

Chaos vs. Harmony

News of Disturbing Events

A galaxy moves toward us,
as ours moves toward it,
relentless as two lovers
who disregard warnings
of the messy disaster
their uncontrolled passions
will set in motion.

The collisions of the suns will rearrange
the Universe. Planets and moons
will fly out of their traditional orbits
turning three-dimensional spirals
into unrecognizable chaos.

Though this will all take place
far into the future, and we will
not be here to see it, news of this
upheaval casts gloom over our small
minds that long for a future
steady and controllable.

Don't worry.
From the beginning of time,
nothing has ever been in control,
except for change and chaos,
out of which comes
the miracles of creation.

A Recurring Dream

The upward mountain road
becomes steeper and narrower,
until my car runs out of room
and plunges off the cliff.

I wake up before I hit bottom.

I'm told that one must hit bottom
before one can change self-
destructive behavior.

Where is bottom?
If I wake up before I hit it,
how will I change?

Life does not promise
a picnic in the park at the end.
The older I get and the narrower my
options, the less I believe I can change.

Bad habits hide in a dark, dusty
closet, ready to emerge and stalk me
as a wolf stalks its prey.

I'm heading for warm sunny meadows.
Why worry about bad habits?
The train is leaving for Priest Point Park.
I'm meeting friends there for a picnic.

Night Riders

A growing dissatisfaction
among a segment of the population
in the town where I live
seeks a way to express itself
by trying out new ways to annoy
the rest of us.

They take the mufflers off their cars
and race the once-quiet streets
from ten p.m. till after midnight.
To make it more annoying,
they schedule breaks between the noise,
just enough to let us would-be sleepers
begin to drift off.

> *Then, they gun those monsters*
> *and wake us up again.*
> *What fun!*

They play that trick with loud fireworks
around Fourth of July, too,
basking in the glee of knowing
that we are cursing them
at three in the morning.

The sirens of the fire trucks
racing to put out grassfires
set by their carelessness,
only adds to the confusion,
and to the pleasure
of the miscreants.

While California Burns

I

Smoke-filled cloud
rides up from California,
engulfs my city. Powdery orange sun
stalls above the western horizon.
No wind disturbs green
leaves of the lotus tree.
People stay behind shut doors.
Stray cat sleeps on my patio.

II

Night's pouring rain
washes the air. Shuddering
rose canes bend down from their
trellis and leaves of the lotus
tree tremble. I stand in the dark
looking out my bathroom
window, see my old neighbor—
collar up, hat pulled down,
scarf around his face—
walk his old black lab.
Ten p.m., as usual.
A car turns down my street,
speeds past, as lucky
cat makes it across in the glare
of heedless headlights.

Robb Elementary

We promised you
before you took your first
breath of life
we would take care of you.

How many arms
reached out to receive you?
As you grew, how many people
in your life riveted
their attention on you,
to keep you safe, to lift you high
so your wings might unfurl
in crackling alignment and fly
to claim the gift of your dreams?

How many stayed awake and vigilant
so you need not fear the tangled
intentions of a troubled soul
who would harm you?
We promised you
our police and our guns would protect you.
No matter what we promised,
when you called for help
your dreams were shot away.

Day of the Election Certification

January 6, 2021

I have sat for hours
eyes glued to the TV,
watching a murderous mob
storm our national Capitol.

I rise from my chair
as if from a bad dream,
stretch tense muscles and look
out my window. The late
afternoon sun hovers
above the horizon. Suddenly,

fast as a gazelle, something
streaks past and out of sight.
Soon it comes back, slower now,
adjusting a slipped headpiece.

It's Olive, my four-year-old
neighbor, dressed as an alligator
and here comes two-year-old
Mosby, in costume as a bee,
bumbling along the sidewalk
beside his father.

It's January, not Halloween,
but they don't care. For them
every day is a day to celebrate.

Questions

On Groundhog Day, February 2, 1936,
I came into this world, on a dark, winter

morning, 3:30 a.m., forming a question:

What am I supposed to do now?

The answer came naturally:

Breathe.

I opened my lungs to the breath of God.
It made me cry.

My birth came between two world wars,
both intended to end all wars.

They didn't.

Now we have power to unleash
a war that could end us all.

How do we extinguish hate
without extinguishing the world?

In our bones we feel infinite
but that is an illusion. We are sad,

lost beings, seeking answers
to questions we're afraid to ask.

We need someone to direct traffic
who knows how to drive.

We need someone who will
look into the future and ask,

> If we keep going like this
> where will we be twenty years from now?

I Want to Learn How to Forgive My Enemies

Not just my own, but the Planet's.
Those who see ubiquitous wildfire smoke
as just smoke, and *not* disintegrated bodies
of trees and birds and animals, and yes,
            people and their homes and livelihoods.

Those who make walking alone dangerous,
            their rage lashing out at the vulnerable.

Those who do not know how to
live with the unknown and who use
            their certainties as a club.

I would like to know how to teach my heart
how to treat the suffering of others
            not as an everyday event, but instead
            as something to mourn and heal.

I go to the aquarium to receive peace from
its quiet solace and think of the creatures
            dying in the ocean's heating waters.

I walk along the stalls of healthful fruits
and vegetables at the Farmer's Market
            and think of children starving
            from lack of nutritious food.

I want to learn how to forgive those who say
            it is meant to be
            that we can do nothing.

I want to learn how to forgive myself
      and to better love
      my friends and my enemies.

What Can I Do?

Tired of the chaos, I don't turn on the news
tonight. It would only bombard me
with scenes of war and desperate
poverty, lies told within a bitter election
campaign, both sides claiming to know
the solution that will save us
from errors made by the other.

I know what I believe yet see my efforts
fail to change the mind of anyone else.
I cannot stop the wars, nor find safety
for those fleeing the bombs.

I cannot find homes for the homeless,
solace for the traumatized,
sanity for the deluded or the disillusioned.
I cannot keep the planet from warming.
I cannot heal my nation's deep divisions.

What can I do?

I can only tend the small patch
of heaven within this body,
plant seeds of love in its soil
and hope they will grow.

The First Worst Year of Forest Fires

Smoke-filled air moves across
state lines and over the sea.
We breath in the particulate
corpses of trees that fall like snow.

Never have we seen such a thing.

We don't let it disturb our daily
lives—unless our own house or town
burns, or asthma tears at our lungs.

This will all go away,
leaving our lives untouched.

We don't look ahead with fear to next year.
We're sure things will be different.

This is only a fluke.

We don't believe what the scientists
tell us, that this is our future to come.

A dense blanket douses the light
and a mournful, orange sun, like a fading ember
descends below the horizon,
while, even in the night, hungry flames
eat Nature's domain and human dwellings,
turning them black and gray—the color of death.

In a World of Social Media

In a world of social media
words form a cacophony of sound.
We become strangers to those

with whom we disagree.
The other becomes our enemy
we perceive across a wide chasm.

I know a man who knew he was dying.
He gathered his family around him,
spoke to them the truth in his heart.

For the first time they saw
his yearning love for them, learned
of his hopes for what they might become.

He spoke of the spiritual
without fear of offending, willed
their discord to become loving harmony.

I know a woman who has a wide
hollow space within her
that weeps no tears.

A space so wide
it can hold the grief of others.
The wider it grows

the more grief it holds
until it contains
the grief of a broken world.

She sings a song of healing
and the grief becomes the song.
The sounds of discord

and grief never go away,
nor does her song of healing
in an alien world of social media.

Meditation on a Foggy Morning

Sky, lakeshore, water
all the same gray mystery.

Four leafless hawthorn trees
organized two by two

and their mirrored reflections
silhouetted in space.

Definition of calm
of silence
of rest after chaos
of losing my bearings
of unbearable loss
of nothingness
of everything I need.

I Love the Gentle Edges of This Day

Turtles warm themselves on a log
along the lakeshore. Songbirds flaunt
new mating garb. Gravel-throated
crows claim their territory.
Rough-ridged tree bark expands
with sap of new growth.

Ornamental trees dance like
ballerinas in dainty pastel tutus
while an orchestra of frogs
in the pond proclaim
the glad rejoicing of Nature.

The caress of April's breeze
opens the eyes of newborn creatures
birthed by the midwife sun.
She slaps them with the breath of life.

Senior Living

Senior Living

I have come here to live
out the end of my life. Does that not
mean I have come here to die?
Someday, not today.

This is a place of memory.
I sit on my balcony in blue
silk revery, recalling the blush
of my twenties, when everything
belonged to the present, my
accomplishments propelled by
promising dreams. Now
what I wish to do accumulates
in piles of undone tasks.

To successfully send a Christmas gift
to a granddaughter and her family
from Harry & David
by using the computer
without help
brings a rare sense of achievement.

Time speeds up, or I slow down.
I look through a narrowing
tunnel to an approaching light
and watch with growing interest
a red-tailed hawk circling above.

Senior Living—A Conversation in the Dining Room

I was in line for a beer
at the Seahawks game, last week.
They wouldn't sell me one without
checking my ID. I was flattered
until they told me
they had to card everyone.

I'm feeling kind of blue today.
My kids finally persuaded me to sell my car.
I won't be driving, anymore.

I know how you feel.
My kids made me sell my car, too.
I was so familiar with the body and fender
man, he was on my speed dial. The last time
I took my car in for the right front
fender, he told me it was mostly Bondo.
He'd have to order a new one.
Better make it two, while you're at it,
I told him.

A little more wine?

Oh, no.
Well, maybe just a little.

Might as well finish up the bottle.

Freedom Lost

I remember the ecstasy
on that day of emancipation
when I got my first driver's license.
I was a vibrant sixteen,
full of hope and seeking adventure.

Now, I take that and feel it backwards—
drab confinement, clipped wings.

Today, I released a part of me,
cut it off like a useless limb.
Today, I gave up my car keys.

How could this happen to me!

Queen of Fourth Floor

Miss C. R. Kitty sleeps on the couch
beside me on a patterned quilt
that sets off her pure, white fur.
Her sleep is so deep
she's not even purring.
I swear she is smiling.

If I stand up, she will awaken
so I sit still in peaceful silence.

What useful thing has she done
today, that deserves such blissful
tranquility?

When I let her out for some exercise,
she paraded down the fourth-floor
halls of this place of retirement,
greeted with a crook of her raised
tail all the friends she met
who stooped to pet her.

In return, she left her white fur
on their black pants as a remembrance.

"Go to the Limits of Your Longing"

—Rainer Maria Rilke, *The Book of Hours*

For what do we long?
A better life? What will make it better?

Assurance of security?
Then, we cut ourselves off
from many of life's possibilities,
build walls to keep out the unexpected.

No pain?
Then, we will not experience growth
that comes from endurance, peace
that comes from healing.

Wealth?
Then, we will not learn the lessons
of doing without, living simply, sharing
with others in mutual need.

Let us long for our source
that gives us breath,
eyes to see flowers and faces of those
we love, ears to hear birdsong and
kind words from friends, a mind
that is grateful for everything that comes—
beauty, terror, and longing itself?

Merging with the Surf

I'm in the mood
for someone possible
to clasp my hand
and run with me
down the sandy beach
meet the rolling surf
fall in with all our life
emerge again
to an ode to joy
and never do we
care about riptide or shark
or anything but possibility
after possibility
and what will come after
we leave the pounding
sound of the water
and its strong grip
on our ankles to whatever
comes from our hands
clasping in a possible way
as we run down
the sandy beach
to our shared joyful
merging with the surf.

Spring Rain Falls After a Long Hesitation

The woods washed and clean
after rain has fallen all day, shines
in the last light of a chemical-
orange and aqua-blue sunset.

The musical splash of ripples
running down the swollen creek
soothes my humming nerves,
clears my mind of negative thoughts.

Water drips like diamonds
from tender tips of newborn leaves.
I lift my face and drink in songs
of birds preparing for night's rest.

Oh, world! How can we not love you more?

I Asked Google

What is the lifespan of a housefly?

Twenty-eight days.

Is that average or optimum?
Is that taking into consideration
the chance of being eaten
midair by a bird,
gobbled in the web of a spider
or struck down by a flyswatter?

And how do they do it?

Die, I mean.
Is time different for them?
Does their twenty-eight days
stretch out, so that it feels
similar to our eighty-five years,
give or take?

Does death come quickly
or does it linger,
taking first the joints
then the organs, and finally, the mind?

Do they know it's coming?
Do they meet it with dread,
or do they consider it a normal
stage of life and succumb graciously?

Do they, as we, treat it as alien?
          *I'm sorry, your questions are beyond
          the scope of my knowledge.*

Image

Sometimes the best of me
gets crowded out by the worst of me
and the quiet voice of sensibility
cannot be heard over the noise
of pride and prejudice.

As a young woman branching out
from the confines of my birthplace
I resisted qualities I might have
inherited from my mother.
I see now, the harder I tried
to shed her influence, the more
it stuck to me like a burr, until
her face confronted me in the mirror.

I don't know when I realized
that I am not alone in wanting
to separate from the one
who gave me birth and,
even after her death, tries
to shape me in her image.

My breath, pouring forth
from the center of my being,
fogs the glass until I see me.

I'm Walking a Tightrope
Holding a Ticking Time-Bomb

How would I live my life if I knew
exactly how many days I had left?

Would I try hard to make every day count
or surrender to fate like a rudderless boat?

Would I seek quiet wonders to enhance my days
or bedazzling thrills?

Would I strive for perfection
or take risks and accept the chance of failure?

Would I wish for more days
or for the end to come sooner?

Would I fill my weird and hungry heart
with longing or with gratitude?

Would I look back on the final day
with satisfaction or regret?

Do I want to know how many days?
I think I'd rather be surprised.

On Employee Appreciation Day:
To the Staff at Wesley Bradley Park

For the things you do for us
        that we used to do ourselves
for your kindness that goes beyond
        your job description
for saying our names in the elevator

for caring for our health
for keeping our apartments clean
for fixing that which is broken
        and changing our lightbulbs

for preparing and serving our food
        and cleaning up after
for preserving our dignity
for protecting our privacy
        and keeping us warm and safe

for keeping us physically fit
for taking us for walks
for setting up for parties
        and providing entertainment
for driving us places we need to go
for your loyalty that brings you to work

please accept this gift of heartfelt gratitude
        because we need you.
We could *not* do without you.

We know it isn't enough.
We know we aren't always easy to please.
We know we make impossible demands.
We know we break your hearts
        sometimes with our pain and our losses.

But where else would you find
        such interesting people
with wacky humor and incredible stories
and who would appreciate you
        as much as we do
when you smile and say our names?

Thank you! Thank you! Thank you!

Predictions

In the new year I'm going
to believe in positive predictions.
Might as well.

Last year, most of us believed
in dire predictions.
All news seemed bad news.
We carried an umbrella wherever
we went, always expecting rain.

Why not believe that sunny days
are right around the corner?
Might as well, since hopes and dreams
can go either way and we never
know which side of the coin
will land up until it is tossed.

I'm going to feel good about
this year and filter out all the depressing
dross, until, come what may,
I end up with days full of laughter and light.
Might as well.

The Secret to Happiness Is:

Don't let it know you are pursuing it.
Pretend you like being unhappy.

Follow at a safe distance, peering
around corners, careful to stay hidden.

If it sees you, pull a sad face and look
the other way. Don't laugh, for heaven's sake.

Tell everyone you meet how miserable you are,
then feel more miserable when they walk away.

Here is the most important part of the secret:
once you have evaded happiness,

once it has forgotten all about you,
for it has not seen you in a long, long time,

sneak up on it. When you get close enough,
grab it. Embrace it. Don't let go.

Why I Think Dave Loves Turtles

You'd think he'd pick a different animal
to love, one more like himself.
Turtles are slow, Dave hurtles ahead
at top speed to capture everything
life has to offer. Sundays,
after the sanctuary doors
close and after the prelude ends,
you see him run up the aisle,
robe flying, a bolt of energy
ready to deliver an electrifying sermon.

After the service, at coffee hour,
surrounded by those who wish to speak
with him, I think he is a little
afraid of the crowd. Afraid they might
love him so much, as with *The Velveteen
Rabbit*, they might rub off his fur.

Does he think then of his turtles,
able, at any moment,
to draw themselves into their shells
where it is safe and peaceful?

He slows down enough
to read a Mary Oliver, Rainer Rilke,
or Rumi poem, enough to absorb meaning
behind every simile and metaphor,
slows down even more to write a poem.

Then, he must stop,
retreat into his carapace,
savor its darkness and silence,
apart from the world's noise and glare.

Though they may not know it,
turtles are poets. I think
that's why Dave loves turtles.

Liberation

I speak too bravely a truth
you don't wish to hear, so you shout,

Be quiet! Stop talking!

This time, I don't take my anger
into my closet and stuff it into the bag
that holds all my other angers,
don't retie its string and set
it back into its dark corner
where I can forget it.

Instead, in a moment of rebellion,
I leave the bag open and set
those forbidden emotions free.

They hop, slither, and fly
out of the bag, making a terrible noise.
Some vanish immediately,
dissipating as if they never existed.
Some stay as my protective allies.

Suddenly, a hush.

Something in the very bottom of the bag
flutters
softly
then, with more force.

Blinking in the light,
out emerges Joy.

She spreads her magnificent
multicolored wings and

flits   flits

          flits

                    in the emancipated air.

Do You Think I Stopped Living Just Because You Did?

Well, you are right. Days and nights
went by with little difference between them.
A hole deep enough to bury the moon
opened in my soul, but then,

the World called and I answered.

I've got to finish this life without you,
fill a new wineskin with new wine,
taste alone a wine glass filled with necessary
action, make decisions by myself, and gather
strength enough to try new possibilities.

In Autumn

In my eighties I've entered autumn
time of harvest, time of loss

my body a dry leaf hanging onto a tree branch.
I see myself diminish, my height

having shrunk three inches. Most of my teeth wear
crowns, scars throughout my body mark

where defective parts are missing. My hair has
lost its color, my eyes their sharp vision

my skin its smooth tautness.
The light slowly changes from summer's glare

to a golden glow deepening into twilight.
It's time to contemplate, recover

my scattered pieces, tend my wounds, cast
off past regrets, anxieties about the future.

In a frantic world full of sorrow and strife,
I have earned the right

to be still, to drift at a leisurely pace and
appear to be wise.

I Shall Not Want

First blush of dawn,
awake from a dream
I don't remember.

The day presents itself
a porcelain cup
waiting to be filled.

Beside still waters
I restore my soul
with poetry, prayer,
and peaceful contemplation.

The rest of the day—
an endless table
of nourishment.

Fragrant tea
overflows my cup.

Our Hero Takes It Slow on a Cloudy Day

The world is not made only of *should*—
that stern-faced word that abides me no slack,
sees no reason for quitting, knows the right
way to make a bed, or gravy without lumps,
insists that I get along with impossible people
who annoy me, and that I must be on time.

There is always room to be a little tardy,
to choose the sweetest pastry, to leave
a bed unmade, until—maybe not today.
Always, I can find time to daydream
about the things I want to do
once I clear those awful *shoulds*
out of my way.

If I Could, I Would Fly You Over the Rainbow

For Karen

Like a monarch butterfly migrating
thousands of miles to a waiting home

or a sheep herded by border collies
to your shepherd's safe sheepfold

or to those places you always wanted to go
but now know you never will

like the bottom of the Grand Canyon
or the top of Mount Kilimanjaro, or to the moon

or to wherever they take coupons for fantastic
dreams, like dyeing your hair purple

or swimming nude in a pool at the base
of a waterfall, or flying high as a kite

or acting in your own movie
with Jack Nicholson as lead.

Someday, over the rainbow
where no pain exists, you'll fly.

The Art of Being a
Healing Presence:
A Guide for Those in
Caring Relationships*

*This thirteen-part poem was written after the ideas from a
booklet by James E. Miller, with Susan C. Cutshall, bearing
the same title, and intended to teach newly ordained deacons
and elders in the Presbyterian denomination.

The Art of Being a Healing Presence

1

Your vision will become clear
only when you can look into your own heart.
Who looks outside, dreams;
who looks inside, awakes.
—Carl Jung

You don't need special training.
Just be available and stay awake.

Someone you know well
or a passing stranger on the street

may require your thoughtful time
or a brief, unexpected moment.

They may need you to keep silent
or speak an affirming word.

Forget about doing it right.
You will learn from your mistakes.

As with any art, the artist
never knows how it will be received.

As with any artist, you must
have courage to put yourself forth.

2

Waking up and staying awake
is hard in a world of distractions.
Your frantic mind struggles to balance
the thousand demands vying for attention.

To awake, you must come to your senses,
be curious, open, not reliving the past,
not inventing the future.

Stop. Look.
Know what is going on
around you and within you.

Quiet your anxious ambition to make
things happen, to influence the outcome.
Stop. Observe.
Let your mindfulness guide you.

Not once, but many times
you must wake yourself.
It's hard to stay awake
when the insistent beat of the world
wants to drive you on.
> *Be effective.*
> *Make a difference.*
> *Keep busy.*

Awake to the beauty of a sunrise,
the miracle of a tree.
Awake to the joys and sorrows
of humanity, to the feelings within yourself.

Awake to the extraordinary
within the ordinary.
Be present to it all.
Awake.

3

You can plant a seed
but you can't make it grow.
That starts within the seed itself.

You can water it, fertilize the soil.
Some say you can foster a plant's
growth by talking to it in a loving way.

Its own intention is to grow.
You are there to encourage it,
affirm its growth.

Neither can you fix people who are broken
or sick. You can plant seeds of healing,
water them with kindness,

nourish them with attentiveness,
but the inclination to be whole
lies within themselves.

Meet them where they are,
listen to their pain, offer your presence,
without expectations.

You may find, when you tend their broken
pieces, you also tend your own.
You also may become more whole.

4

You can search the ten-fold universe
and not find a single being more worthy
of loving kindness than yourself.
—*Buddha*

Only after you have looked within,
offered your own jagged pieces for healing
will you be a healing presence to someone else.

Only after you have walked through
the darkness within yourself,
can you offer a light to guide
another through their darkness.

Not that you may ever be completely healed
or have no dark places left within you.
You are what you are.
Accept and love your humanness,
so you allow others
to accept and love their own.

5

Create within yourself a sanctuary,
a calm place where others may
come and safely be themselves,
honest and open,
trusting and free.

Place any stress you carry
in the palm of your open hand
and let it fly away.

6

To be a healing presence
there is no up or down
no less or more
no holy versus profane
no benefactor or obliged.

There is only respect and dignity
worth and wholeness

        and love

for yourself and the other

7

Listen
     So they know you care
          so they know they have value
               so they feel empowered and free

Hold them
     in your thoughts throughout the day
          as part of your spiritual practice
               in your embrace, if they need or want it

Talk
     less than you listen
          Respond to their talk
               Reveal your own story, only if called

Let silence
     make room for deeper healing
          Let it bring comfort
               Hear what the silence is saying

Be still
     Quiet your body
          Focus your eyes on the one who needs healing
               Feel your body's sensations
                    that they may lead you

Be your natural self
     Follow your instincts
          Trust your intuition
               Lead the other to a centered place

Receive
    what comes, with an open mind
        Accept what the other has to say
            Embrace what the experience offers

8

When they have lost hope—
    hope for them.
When they no longer believe—
    believe for them.
When they can no longer lift themselves up—
    reach out your hand.

9

Be near me when my light is low.
—Alfred Lord Tennyson

Plenty of people can tell those
in need what they could do to feel better.
Plenty of strong people,
seeing weakness, can offer
superior wisdom. They know
just what will fix them.

What those who feel lousy need
is for someone who *doesn't*
know all the answers to sit by
and listen to their story.

10

When the aged can no longer live
on their own, they are set in place,
like books on library shelves.
Enter there with reverence.
These books are full of stories
needing to be read.

Approach with care. They may be wary
that you are not able to accept
what they have to lay before you.
They may fear you will leave, distressed
by their situation, and never return.

Are you able to look at swollen legs
so timidly revealed,
skin cracked and weeping?
Can you affirm pain and fear
with a face full of empathy and love,
without a trace of your own fear?
Can you accept when they know
their end is near and still
celebrate with them
this day that they still live?

Are you able to walk away
buoyed by their courage and endurance,
wanting to come back to hear
more of their precious stories?
Are you willing to feel their pain
without being consumed by it,
to allow love to build
without a fear of loss?

Then, you may enter into their space
as a healing presence, and come away,
fully yourself and whole.

11

What will you gain
through the art of being?

You will learn to live
more fully in the moment,
claim your days and live them well,
knowing they are precious.

You will meet your genuine self,
make it more available to others.

You will be more open
to others' heart stories
in a way that will build you up.

You will learn gratitude
from receiving others' gratitude
for what you have given them.

12

After you had taken your leave,
I found God's footprints on the floor.
—Rabindranath Tagore

The healing presence moves us
into the realm of sacredness,
where life is messy and mysterious,
weary and wonderful,
exasperating and joyful.

Sacredness reveals itself from
where it's been hiding and we
haven't thought to look.
We see with new eyes
pain and death straight on,
and know that they are sacred, too.

Let us seek the sacred in our
everyday lives, and when
we gather with others to worship.
Let us seek it through the arts,
through acts of justice,
when we plant a garden,
take a walk in the woods,
and when we lend our healing presence
to someone who needs it.

13

And we are put on earth a little space
that we might learn to bear the beams of love.
—William Blake

The art of being will transform you.
It will come, not from you, but through you,
to all those around you. Let it ripple out
in simplicity, and in gratitude.

Be willing to just be.

Acknowledgments

The author thanks and acknowledges the publishers of the following collections where some of these poems previously appeared:

Author's Books

Shapes of Time (MoonPath Press, 2022): "When Things Happen Unexpectedly," "Depression," "All Things Must End," "Day of the Election Certification," "In Autumn"

Thresholds (MoonPath Press, 2017): "New Friend," "Affliction," "When I Fly"

Anthologies

7 Secrets to Happiness in 7 Minutes, Compiled by Lana Hechtman Ayers (Night Rain Press, 2024): "The Secret to Happiness Is:"

Filling the Cracks with Gold: Writing Inspired by James Crews' Poem "Small Moments," Compiled by Lana Hechtman Ayers (Night Rain Press, 2024): "Our Hero Takes It Slow on a Cloudy Day"

Women Writing: On the Edge of Dark and Light, A compilation of Catherine Place Poets (Pilgrim Spirit Communications, 2015): "New Friend"

Gratitude

My heartfelt gratitude to:

the Senate and the Congress, who recently passed the National Plan to End Parkinson's Act,

and to President Biden, who signed it, which will unite the federal government and private enterprise in a mission to prevent and find a cure for PD, and provide financial aid in the treatment of those living with PD;

those organizations working to aid and educate those living with Parkinson's, such as American Parkinson's Association, Northwest Parkinson's Foundation, Michael J. Fox Foundation, and Davis Phinney Foundation;

the many who have contributed financially to the cause of Parkinson's;

the researchers and those who sign up as research "lab rats";

those in the medical field, who treat the various symptoms of Parkinson's;

the caregivers, bless their hearts;

those brave warriors living with Parkinson's, who lead by their example and give the rest of us courage to make the best out of every day we live;

and Chelsea Beck, who leads a class every Tuesday and Thursday for those with PD, where we learn voice training, memory games, big movement, multitasking, balance, and more.

Also, to Debra Elisa and Sharon Carter, who read my work and responded generously for the cover;

all my friends in my poetry groups on Zoom, who keep me writing;

my friends at Wesley Bradley Park senior community, and Immanuel Presbyterian Church, who give me reason to write;

my beloved family, who enhance my life;

and Lana Hechtman Ayers, without whose encouragement
and mentorship this book would not exist.

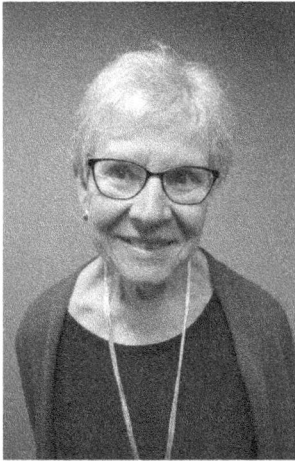

About the Author

Like Joy is Glenna Cook's third full-length collection of poems, all published by MoonPath Press. The first is *Thresholds* (2017), a finalist for the Washington State Book Award for Poetry in 2018. The second is *Shapes of Time* (2022).

Cook grew up in Olympia, Washington, where, at age 18, she married her husband, Kenneth. They had 3 children (their oldest, a son, died of cancer in 2016 at age 60), and she has 9 grandchildren and 8 great-grandchildren. After a 25-year career with the telephone company, she retired from US West Communications in 1990, then immediately enrolled in college. She graduated from the University of Puget Sound, Magna cum Laude in 1994 at age 58, with a BA in English Literature. While at university, she won the Hearst Essay Prize for the Humanities and the Nixeon Civille Handy Prize in poetry. She is a Hedgebrook alumna and a member of Phi Kappa Phi Honor Society.

She has read her poetry many places in the Puget Sound region, and published dozens of poems in journals and anthologies, the latest being *This Light Called Darkness*, a Raven Chronicles anthology (2023), and *When a Woman Tells the Truth: Writings and Creative Work by Women Over 80*, edited by Dena Taylor and Wilma Marcus Chandler (2024).

Her husband died in 2018, after 63 years of marriage. Cook has Parkinson's disease, which she keeps at bay with medicine, diet, and a rigorous exercise program. She serves as an advocate for others with Parkinson's disease. She loves reading, watching PBS and Netflix, taking walks, and interacting with people. Two of her favorite sayings are: *We make our own weather*, and (from Rumi) *What you seek is seeking you.*

www.ingramcontent.com/pod-product-compliance
Lightning Source LLC
Chambersburg PA
CBHW022101020426
42335CB00012B/782